30-Minute Meal Prep: Quick and Healthy Recipes for Busy People"

An introduction to meal prep and its benefits for health and time management.

Acknowledgments

I would like to express my deepest gratitude to all those who made this book possible.

First, I want to thank my family and friends for their unwavering support throughout this journey. Your encouragement and belief in me have been a constant source of motivation.

A special thank you to my readers—those passionate about healthy eating and time management. You inspire me to create practical content that can help simplify your daily life while maintaining a balanced lifestyle.

To the community of health enthusiasts, meal preppers, and nutrition experts who generously share their knowledge, thank you for fostering an environment of growth and inspiration.

Lastly, I would like to thank my dedicated team and the professionals who contributed to the development of this book. Your expertise, guidance, and attention to detail have been invaluable.

This book is as much yours as it is mine.

Thank you!

Table of Contents

Introduction

Chapter 1: What is Meal Prep?

Chapter 2: Getting Started with Meal Prep

Chapter 3: Nutrition Basics for Meal Prep

- Understanding Macronutrients (Proteins, Carbs, Fats)
- Balancing Nutrients in Your Meal Plan
- Portion Control and Serving Sizes
- Tips for Keeping Meals Nutritious and Delicious

Chapter 4: Breakfast Recipes in 30 Minutes or Less

- Quick and Nutritious Smoothies
- Make-Ahead Breakfast Bowls
- Healthy Overnight Oats Recipes
- Easy Egg-Based Dishes for Busy Mornings

Chapter 5: Lunch Recipes for On-The-Go

- Simple Salads That Last All Week
- Hearty Sandwiches and Wraps
- One-Pot Pasta and Rice Dishes
- Mason Jar Meals for Easy Transportation

Chapter 6: Dinner Recipes for Weeknight Ease

- Fast and Flavorful Stir-Fries
- Sheet Pan Meals for Easy Clean-Up
- Healthy 30-Minute Soups and Stews
- Quick Protein and Vegetable Combinations

Chapter 7: Snacks and Side Dishes

- Healthy Snacks for Work or School
- Easy Sides to Compliment Any Meal
- Snack Prep Ideas for Busy Weeks
- Storing and Packing Snacks for Maximum Freshness

Chapter 8: Batch Cooking for Meal Prep

- What is Batch Cooking?
- How to Batch Cook Efficiently
- Best Batch Cooking Recipes
- Freezing and Storing Batch-Cooked Meals

Chapter 9: Time-Saving Tips for Meal Prep

- How to Optimize Your Meal Prep Time
- Strategies for Multi-Tasking in the Kitchen
- Organizing Your Fridge and Pantry for Efficiency
- Prepping Multiple Meals at Once

Chapter 10: Meal Prep for Weight Loss and Fitness

- Tailoring Your Meal Prep to Your Fitness Goals
- High-Protein Meal Prep Recipes

Chapter 11: Vegetarian and Vegan Meal Prep Ideas

Chapter 12: Long-Term Meal Prep Success

Conclusion

Resources

Chapter 1: What is Meal Prep?

Definition of Meal Prep

Meal prep, short for meal preparation, refers to the process of planning, preparing, and organizing meals in advance. It typically involves cooking food in batches and portioning it out for consumption over a period of time, usually a few days or a week. This approach allows you to have ready-to-eat meals or components that require minimal preparation before serving. Whether it's chopping vegetables, cooking grains, or preparing entire dishes, meal prep helps to save time, reduce daily stress, and ensure that healthy meals are always accessible.

Why Meal Prep is Important for a Busy Lifestyle

In today's fast-paced world, finding time to cook fresh, healthy meals every day can be challenging. Between work, family obligations, and personal activities, many people turn to unhealthy fast food or processed meals because they are convenient. However, meal prepping allows you to avoid these pitfalls. By setting aside a specific time to prepare your meals for the week, you eliminate the need to make last-minute food choices, which are often less nutritious. Meal prep not only saves time but also helps ensure that your meals align with your health and wellness goals.

Key Benefits of Meal Prep (Health, Time, and Money)

Meal prep offers several key benefits that make it a valuable habit for anyone trying to maintain a busy schedule while eating well:

- Health: By preparing meals ahead of time, you have full control over the ingredients, ensuring that your food is balanced and nutritious. This makes it easier to avoid excessive sugar, salt, and unhealthy fats often found in takeout and processed foods.
- Time: Meal prep reduces the amount of time you spend cooking each day. Instead of scrambling to prepare a fresh meal after a long day, you simply need to reheat a pre-cooked dish or assemble pre-chopped ingredients into a quick meal.
- Money: Planning your meals ahead allows you to create a shopping list and stick to it, which helps reduce impulse buys and food waste. You're also less likely to rely on expensive takeout or restaurant meals when you already have food ready to eat.

Common Myths About Meal Prep

Despite its numerous advantages, there are several misconceptions about meal prep that often prevent people from getting started. Let's dispel a few of the most common myths:

- "Meal prep takes too much time."
  While it's true that meal prepping requires some upfront effort, the time saved throughout the week far outweighs the initial investment. With practice, you can prep several days' worth of meals in just a few hours.
- "It's boring to eat the same thing every day."
  Many people believe that meal prep means eating the same dish for multiple meals. However, with variety in ingredients and cooking methods, meal prepping can offer diverse and exciting options throughout the week. Prepping meal components like proteins, grains, and vegetables allows you to mix and match for different meals.
- "Meal prep is only for fitness enthusiasts."
  While meal prep is popular among people with specific fitness or weight loss goals, it's not just for athletes or bodybuilders. Anyone who wants to eat healthier, save time, and reduce stress in the kitchen can benefit from meal prep.

Chapter 2: Getting Started with Meal Prep

Essential Kitchen Tools and Equipment

Before diving into meal prep, it's important to have the right tools and equipment. A well-stocked kitchen will make the process faster and more efficient. Here's a list of essential items that will help you prepare meals with ease:

- Sharp Knives: A good chef's knife and paring knife are indispensable for chopping vegetables, fruits, and meats quickly and safely.
- Cutting Boards: Use separate cutting boards for meats and vegetables to avoid cross-contamination. Opt for a durable, easy-to-clean board.
- Measuring Cups and Spoons: Accurate measurements ensure consistent portions and recipe success, especially when following meal plans.
- Mixing Bowls: Multiple mixing bowls of different sizes will help you prep ingredients, mix salads, or marinate proteins.
- Food Containers: Airtight containers are essential for storing prepped meals. Choose BPA-free plastic or glass containers that can be microwaved, frozen, and transported easily.
- Sheet Pans and Baking Dishes: These are perfect for roasting vegetables, baking proteins, or preparing one-pan meals that save on time and cleanup.
- Slow Cooker or Instant Pot: These appliances are meal prep lifesavers. They allow you to cook large quantities of food with minimal effort, perfect for batch cooking.
- Blender or Food Processor: For smoothies, sauces, or chopping ingredients quickly, a blender or food processor can be incredibly useful.

With these tools in your kitchen, you'll be ready to tackle meal prep like a pro!

Must-Have Ingredients for a Well-Stocked Pantry

A well-stocked pantry is key to successful meal prep. Having versatile ingredients on hand allows you to create a variety of meals without running to the store constantly. Here's a list of must-have pantry staples:

- Grains: Brown rice, quinoa, oats, whole-wheat pasta, and couscous are versatile, nutrient-dense carbs that can be used in many meals.
- Canned Goods: Keep canned beans (like black beans, chickpeas, and lentils) for quick protein, as well as canned tomatoes for sauces, soups, and stews.

- Spices and Seasonings: Salt, pepper, garlic powder, paprika, cumin, turmeric, and herbs like oregano and thyme are essential for adding flavor to your dishes.
- Oils and Vinegars: Olive oil, coconut oil, apple cider vinegar, and balsamic vinegar are great for cooking and dressing salads.
- Nuts and Seeds: Almonds, walnuts, chia seeds, and flaxseeds are excellent sources of healthy fats and protein. They can be added to salads, smoothies, or used as snacks.
- Frozen Vegetables: Frozen vegetables are a convenient and budget-friendly way to add nutrients to your meals when fresh produce isn't available.
- Proteins: Stock your fridge and freezer with lean meats like chicken breast, turkey, and fish, as well as plant-based proteins like tofu and tempeh.

With these ingredients, you'll have a solid foundation to create nutritious and varied meals each week.

How to Plan Your First Meal Prep

Getting started with meal prep can feel overwhelming, but with a simple plan in place, it becomes much more manageable. Here's how to plan your first meal prep:

1. Set a Goal: Determine how many meals you want to prep. Are you planning meals for the entire week, or just a few days? Knowing this will help you plan your portions and grocery list accordingly.
2. Choose Simple Recipes: Start with easy-to-make recipes that require minimal ingredients. Think about meals that you already enjoy and can scale up for batch cooking. Aim for dishes that include a protein, a carb, and a vegetable.
3. Create a Grocery List: Once you've chosen your recipes, write down all the ingredients you need. Stick to the list while shopping to avoid impulse buys and stay on budget.
4. Set Aside Prep Time: Dedicate a specific day and time for meal prep. Many people choose Sundays, but pick a time that works best for your schedule. Block off 2-3 hours for prepping, cooking, and cleaning up.
5. Prepping and Storing: Cook your meals, portion them out into individual containers, and label them if necessary. Store them in the fridge or freezer, depending on how soon you'll be eating them.

By following these simple steps, you'll be able to prep several meals in a short period, ensuring you're ready for the week ahead.

Beginner Mistakes to Avoid

As with any new habit, there are some common mistakes that beginners make when starting meal prep. Here are a few to watch out for:

- Overcomplicating Recipes: Keep things simple at the beginning. Avoid recipes with too many ingredients or complicated cooking techniques. Start with basics and build your confidence as you go.
- Not Prepping Enough Variety: While batch cooking is convenient, prepping the same meal for the entire week can get monotonous. Try to mix and match ingredients or rotate meals every few days to keep things interesting.
- Underestimating Portions: Be mindful of portion sizes, especially if you're prepping for weight loss or fitness goals. Use measuring cups or a kitchen scale to ensure your portions are aligned with your goals.
- Not Storing Food Properly: Improper storage can lead to spoiled food or soggy meals. Make sure your containers are airtight and store perishable items in the fridge or freezer to maintain freshness.
- Skipping the Prep Plan: Don't go into meal prep without a plan. Skipping steps like making a grocery list or setting aside time for prep can lead to stress and disorganization, making meal prep feel more like a burden than a time-saver.

By avoiding these common pitfalls, you'll be able to streamline your meal prep process and enjoy the benefits of having ready-made, healthy meals at your fingertips.

Chapter 3: Nutrition Basics for Meal Prep

Understanding Macronutrients (Proteins, Carbs, Fats)
When it comes to meal prep, understanding the three key macronutrients—proteins, carbohydrates, and fats—is essential for creating balanced, nutritious meals. These nutrients provide your body with the energy and components it needs to function properly.

- **Proteins**: Proteins are the building blocks of your muscles, organs, and tissues. They play a critical role in repair and recovery, making them especially important for active individuals. Common sources of protein include chicken, turkey, beef, fish, eggs, tofu, beans, and lentils.

- **Carbohydrates**: Carbs are your body's main source of energy. They are broken down into glucose, which fuels your brain and muscles. Healthy carb sources include whole grains (like brown rice and quinoa), sweet potatoes, oats, fruits, and vegetables. Focus on complex carbohydrates, as they provide longer-lasting energy and are rich in fiber.
- **Fats**: Fats help absorb vitamins, provide energy, and support cell function. Healthy fats, such as those found in avocados, nuts, seeds, and olive oil, are essential for heart and brain health. Avoid trans fats and limit saturated fats, which can negatively impact your health.

Understanding how to balance these macronutrients in your meals will help you create satisfying dishes that keep you energized throughout the day.

Balancing Nutrients in Your Meal Plan

A balanced meal plan includes the right proportion of macronutrients to meet your body's needs. While the specific ratio of proteins, carbs, and fats may vary depending on your goals (such as weight loss, muscle gain, or overall health), a general guideline is the **"plate method"**:

- **Half of your plate** should consist of non-starchy vegetables like leafy greens, broccoli, bell peppers, or carrots. These vegetables are nutrient-dense and low in calories, making them a great base for most meals.
- **A quarter of your plate** should be protein. Choose lean proteins like chicken, fish, tofu, or legumes for a healthy option that keeps you full and supports muscle repair.
- **The remaining quarter of your plate** should be made up of whole grains or starchy vegetables like brown rice, quinoa, sweet potatoes, or whole-grain pasta. These provide long-lasting energy and essential fiber.

In addition, include a small portion of healthy fats, like olive oil for cooking or a handful of nuts added to salads or snacks. The goal is to create balanced meals that offer a variety of nutrients, while controlling portion sizes to prevent overeating.

Portion Control and Serving Sizes

One of the advantages of meal prep is that it allows you to control your portion sizes, which is especially important if you're trying to manage your weight or adhere to specific dietary goals. Here are some guidelines for portion control:

- **Protein**: A serving of protein should be about the size of your palm (roughly 3-4 ounces for meats or fish). Plant-based proteins, like beans or lentils, can be measured as half a cup per serving.

- **Carbohydrates**: For grains or starchy vegetables, aim for a portion about the size of a cupped hand, or approximately half a cup. For more fibrous vegetables like leafy greens, you can increase the portion to fill half your plate.
- **Fats**: Healthy fats are calorie-dense, so it's important to watch portion sizes. A thumb-sized portion of oils, butter, or avocado (around one tablespoon) is generally sufficient per meal.

Using measuring tools like cups, spoons, or even a kitchen scale when portioning out your meals during prep can help ensure you're not overeating and keeping your meals aligned with your goals.

Tips for Keeping Meals Nutritious and Delicious

Maintaining the balance between nutrition and flavor is key to enjoying your meal prep. Here are some simple tips to make sure your meals are both healthy and delicious:

- **Use Fresh Herbs and Spices**: Herbs and spices not only add flavor but also pack powerful antioxidants and nutrients. Experiment with garlic, ginger, cilantro, basil, turmeric, and cumin to give your meals depth without adding extra calories.
- **Healthy Cooking Methods**: Opt for grilling, baking, steaming, or stir-frying instead of deep-frying. These cooking methods allow you to retain the natural flavors of your ingredients while keeping meals light and nutritious.
- **Incorporate a Variety of Colors**: Eating a variety of colorful vegetables ensures you're getting a wide range of vitamins and minerals. Plus, visually appealing meals are more satisfying and exciting to eat.
- **Add Healthy Fats**: Instead of relying on heavy dressings or sauces, incorporate healthy fats like avocado, nuts, seeds, or olive oil. These add richness and texture to your meals, keeping them filling and flavorful.
- **Be Mindful of Salt and Sugar**: While salt enhances flavor, too much can lead to water retention and high blood pressure. Use it sparingly and experiment with other seasonings. Similarly, avoid adding excessive sugar to sauces or marinades—natural sweeteners like honey or maple syrup can be used in moderation.

By following these tips, you'll create meals that are not only good for you but also enjoyable to eat every day.

Chapter 4: Breakfast Recipes in 30 Minutes or Less

Quick and Nutritious Smoothies

Smoothies are the ultimate quick breakfast option. They are nutritious, versatile, and can be made in just minutes. Here are a few ideas for smoothie combinations that are both delicious and packed with essential nutrients:

- **Green Power Smoothie**: Combine spinach, frozen mango, a banana, and a scoop of protein powder with unsweetened almond milk. Blend until smooth for a nutrient-packed start to your day.
- **Berry Antioxidant Smoothie**: Blend mixed berries (strawberries, blueberries, raspberries) with Greek yogurt, a tablespoon of chia seeds, and a splash of water or almond milk for a smoothie rich in antioxidants and fiber.
- **Peanut Butter Banana Smoothie**: For a filling and protein-rich breakfast, blend a frozen banana with a tablespoon of peanut butter, a scoop of protein powder, and almond milk. This smoothie is perfect for post-workout recovery.
- **Tropical Sunshine Smoothie**: Blend frozen pineapple, mango, coconut water, and a tablespoon of flaxseeds for a refreshing and hydrating smoothie with a tropical twist.

Smoothies can be made even faster by prepping the ingredients in advance. Store individual smoothie ingredients in freezer-safe bags so all you need to do is dump and blend in the morning.

Make-Ahead Breakfast Bowls

Breakfast bowls are another easy way to ensure you're starting your day with a healthy, filling meal. These bowls can be prepped in advance and stored in the fridge for quick assembly during the week. Here are some ideas:

- **Quinoa and Veggie Breakfast Bowl**: Cook a batch of quinoa and store it in the fridge. In the morning, top the quinoa with sautéed spinach, cherry tomatoes, avocado slices, and a poached egg for a savory breakfast bowl full of protein and fiber.
- **Greek Yogurt and Granola Bowl**: Layer Greek yogurt, fresh berries, and a handful of homemade or store-bought granola. Add a drizzle of honey or a sprinkle of chia seeds for an extra nutrient boost.
- **Sweet Potato and Black Bean Breakfast Bowl**: Roast sweet potato cubes in advance and combine them with black beans, scrambled eggs, and a sprinkle of cheese. Top with salsa or avocado for a Southwest-inspired breakfast bowl.
- **Overnight Oats Breakfast Bowl**: Combine oats, almond milk, chia seeds, and your choice of toppings (like nuts, fruit, or honey) the night before. In the morning, you'll have a hearty and delicious breakfast waiting for you.

These breakfast bowls are easy to adapt based on what you have on hand, making them a flexible and nutritious option for busy mornings.

Healthy Overnight Oats Recipes

Overnight oats are the perfect make-ahead breakfast option. Simply combine oats with liquid and let them sit in the fridge overnight. By morning, they'll be soft and ready to eat. Here are some tasty variations to try:

- **Classic Overnight Oats**: Combine rolled oats with your choice of milk (almond, soy, or regular) and a spoonful of chia seeds. Sweeten with honey or maple syrup and top with fresh berries for a classic, balanced breakfast.
- **Chocolate Peanut Butter Overnight Oats**: For a decadent yet healthy breakfast, mix oats with unsweetened almond milk, a tablespoon of cocoa powder, and a spoonful of peanut butter. Top with a sprinkle of dark chocolate chips for a sweet touch.
- **Apple Cinnamon Overnight Oats**: Mix oats with almond milk and a dash of cinnamon. Add chopped apples and a drizzle of honey for a sweet, fiber-rich breakfast. This can also be topped with walnuts for extra crunch and omega-3s.
- **Banana Nut Overnight Oats**: Combine oats with almond milk, mashed banana, and a tablespoon of almond butter. Add chia seeds or flaxseeds for added nutrients, and top with sliced almonds for a nutty, delicious breakfast.

Overnight oats are not only time-efficient but also endlessly customizable, allowing you to switch up flavors and toppings based on your preferences.

Easy Egg-Based Dishes for Busy Mornings

Eggs are a versatile, protein-packed breakfast option that can be cooked in advance for quick assembly during the week. Here are a few easy egg-based dishes you can meal prep for busy mornings:

- **Egg Muffins**: Whisk eggs with your choice of veggies (like spinach, bell peppers, and onions) and pour the mixture into a muffin tin. Add a sprinkle of cheese and bake until set. Store these egg muffins in the fridge for up to five days, reheating them as needed for a quick breakfast.
- **Scrambled Egg Breakfast Burritos**: Make a large batch of scrambled eggs and combine them with sautéed vegetables, black beans, and cheese. Wrap the mixture in whole-wheat tortillas and freeze them individually. In the morning, just pop a burrito in the microwave for a hearty, on-the-go meal.
- **Veggie-Packed Frittata**: A frittata is an easy way to prepare eggs for multiple meals. Whisk eggs with a variety of vegetables (like mushrooms, zucchini, and tomatoes), pour the mixture into an oven-safe skillet, and bake until the eggs are set. Slice the frittata into portions and store in the fridge for quick breakfasts.
- **Avocado Toast with Poached Eggs**: For a quick breakfast, toast whole-grain bread and top it with mashed avocado. Poach or fry an egg and place it on top of the toast for a balanced meal rich in healthy fats and protein.

These egg-based dishes are filling, nutritious, and perfect for making ahead, allowing you to enjoy a high-protein breakfast even on your busiest mornings.

Chapter 5: Lunch Recipes in 30 Minutes or Less

Healthy Grain Bowls

Grain bowls are a versatile and balanced lunch option that can be prepped in advance and customized to your taste. By combining whole grains, lean proteins, healthy fats, and vegetables, you can create a nutritious meal that's quick and easy to prepare. Here are a few combinations to get you started:

- **Mediterranean Quinoa Bowl**: Start with cooked quinoa as your base. Add chopped cucumbers, cherry tomatoes, red onions, and Kalamata olives. Top with crumbled feta cheese, grilled chicken, and a drizzle of olive oil and lemon juice. This bowl is rich in protein and healthy fats, making it a satisfying and flavorful lunch.
- **Mexican-Inspired Brown Rice Bowl**: Use brown rice as your base and add black beans, grilled corn, avocado slices, and diced tomatoes. Top with shredded chicken or beef and a sprinkle of cheddar cheese. Finish with a dollop of salsa or Greek yogurt for a zesty, protein-packed meal.
- **Teriyaki Salmon and Veggie Bowl**: Cook a serving of brown rice or farro and top it with grilled or baked salmon. Add steamed broccoli, snap peas, and sliced carrots. Drizzle with a homemade teriyaki sauce (made from soy sauce, honey, garlic, and ginger) for a delicious, nutrient-rich meal.
- **Falafel and Couscous Bowl**: Prepare whole-wheat couscous and top it with homemade or store-bought falafel, hummus, cucumber slices, and cherry tomatoes. Drizzle with tahini sauce for a Middle Eastern-inspired lunch that's rich in plant-based protein and fiber.

Grain bowls are ideal for meal prep because you can prepare large batches of grains, proteins, and vegetables in advance, then assemble the bowls when you're ready to eat.

Hearty Salads that Stay Fresh

Salads are a great lunch option for anyone looking to stay light yet satisfied during the day. The key to a great meal prep salad is ensuring it stays fresh and doesn't become soggy. Here are some hearty salad ideas that hold up well for meal prep:

- **Chopped Kale and Quinoa Salad**: Kale is a sturdy green that holds up well in the fridge, making it perfect for meal prep. Massage the kale with olive oil and lemon juice to soften it, then mix in cooked quinoa, roasted sweet potatoes, chickpeas, and feta cheese. This salad is packed with fiber, vitamins, and plant-based protein.
- **Chicken Caesar Salad with a Twist**: Use Romaine lettuce or a blend of hearty greens as the base. Top with grilled chicken breast, homemade or store-bought croutons, and

shaved Parmesan cheese. Instead of a heavy Caesar dressing, try a lighter Greek yogurt-based version to keep the salad healthy and fresh.

- **Asian Sesame Cabbage Salad**: Combine shredded green and purple cabbage with carrots, bell peppers, and edamame. Toss with grilled chicken or shrimp and top with sesame seeds. Use a simple sesame-ginger dressing (made with soy sauce, rice vinegar, sesame oil, and ginger) to add flavor without overpowering the freshness of the vegetables.
- **Greek Chickpea Salad**: This salad uses chickpeas as the base for a filling, protein-rich meal. Add diced cucumbers, cherry tomatoes, red onion, Kalamata olives, and feta cheese. Drizzle with olive oil and lemon juice. This salad stores well for several days and makes for a quick, refreshing lunch.

The key to successful salad meal prep is to store the dressing separately and add it just before serving. This keeps the salad fresh and crunchy.

Wraps and Sandwiches for On-the-Go

Wraps and sandwiches are classic lunchtime staples that are easy to make, portable, and customizable. Here are some healthy variations that go beyond the basic sandwich:

- **Turkey and Avocado Wrap**: Use a whole-wheat or spinach wrap and layer slices of turkey breast, mashed avocado, spinach, and a slice of tomato. Add a drizzle of mustard or hummus for extra flavor. This wrap is a great source of lean protein and healthy fats.
- **Chicken Caesar Wrap**: Toss grilled chicken breast with a light Caesar dressing and wrap it up with Romaine lettuce and Parmesan cheese in a whole-wheat tortilla. This wrap delivers all the flavors of a Caesar salad in a convenient, hand-held form.
- **Veggie and Hummus Wrap**: Spread hummus on a whole-wheat wrap and add sliced cucumbers, bell peppers, shredded carrots, and spinach. For added protein, include a few slices of avocado or some crumbled feta cheese. This wrap is packed with fiber, vitamins, and plant-based protein.
- **Tuna Salad Sandwich**: Mix canned tuna with Greek yogurt, lemon juice, and diced celery for a healthier take on traditional tuna salad. Serve it on whole-grain bread with lettuce and tomato for a quick, protein-rich lunch.

Wraps and sandwiches can be prepared the night before or even a few days in advance, making them a go-to option for busy weeks.

One-Pan Lunches for Easy Clean-Up

One-pan meals are perfect for those who want a quick, fuss-free lunch that requires minimal clean-up. Here are some easy one-pan lunch ideas that you can prepare in just 30 minutes:

- **Sheet Pan Chicken and Vegetables**: Toss chicken breasts or thighs with olive oil, garlic, and your favorite spices. Add sliced bell peppers, zucchini, and red onion. Spread everything out on a baking sheet and roast at 400°F for 20-25 minutes. Serve with a side of quinoa or brown rice for a complete meal.

- **Baked Salmon and Asparagus**: Place salmon fillets on a sheet pan and drizzle with olive oil, lemon juice, and garlic. Add asparagus spears to the pan and season with salt and pepper. Bake for 15-20 minutes until the salmon is cooked through and the asparagus is tender. This is a simple, low-carb meal that's rich in omega-3s and vitamins.
- **Sweet Potato and Black Bean Tacos**: Roast diced sweet potatoes with cumin and chili powder on a sheet pan. Once cooked, serve them in whole-wheat tortillas with black beans, shredded lettuce, and salsa for a quick and healthy taco lunch.
- **Roasted Vegetable and Farro Bowl**: Roast a variety of vegetables (such as Brussels sprouts, carrots, and sweet potatoes) with olive oil and balsamic vinegar. Once roasted, serve them over cooked farro and top with a sprinkle of goat cheese or a drizzle of tahini for a filling and nutritious lunch.

One-pan lunches are not only easy to prepare but also perfect for batch cooking. You can make multiple servings at once and store them for later in the week.

Chapter 6: Dinner Recipes in 30 Minutes or Less

Quick Stir-Fry Dishes

Stir-fry meals are a great way to create healthy, well-balanced dinners in just a few minutes. By using a variety of vegetables, lean proteins, and flavorful sauces, you can have a satisfying meal on the table in no time. Here are some easy stir-fry ideas:

- **Chicken and Broccoli Stir-Fry**: Heat a tablespoon of oil in a large skillet or wok and cook sliced chicken breast until browned. Add broccoli florets, garlic, and a touch of soy sauce. Stir-fry for 5-7 minutes until the chicken is fully cooked and the broccoli is tender. Serve over brown rice or quinoa for a complete meal.
- **Beef and Snow Pea Stir-Fry**: Thinly slice beef sirloin or flank steak and cook in a hot skillet with sesame oil. Add snow peas, bell peppers, and sliced onions. Toss with a homemade stir-fry sauce made from soy sauce, ginger, garlic, and honey. This meal is packed with protein and fiber, and the sweet and savory flavors make it extra delicious.
- **Tofu and Vegetable Stir-Fry**: For a vegetarian option, cube firm tofu and stir-fry it with vegetables like zucchini, bell peppers, and snap peas. Use a simple sauce made from soy sauce, rice vinegar, and a touch of Sriracha for heat. This plant-based dinner is quick, nutritious, and filling.
- **Shrimp and Bok Choy Stir-Fry**: Stir-fry shrimp with garlic and ginger until pink, then add chopped bok choy and mushrooms. Toss with soy sauce and sesame oil for a light yet flavorful dinner. Serve with a side of steamed jasmine rice for a complete meal in under 30 minutes.

Stir-frying is fast, easy, and a great way to use up any leftover vegetables in your fridge.

Sheet Pan Dinners for Easy Clean-Up

Sheet pan dinners are ideal for busy weeknights because they require minimal prep and clean-up. Simply arrange your ingredients on a baking sheet, roast them in the oven, and dinner is ready. Here are some tasty sheet pan dinner ideas:

- **Lemon Garlic Chicken with Vegetables**: Arrange chicken thighs, sliced carrots, and red potatoes on a baking sheet. Drizzle with olive oil, lemon juice, and minced garlic. Season with salt, pepper, and rosemary, then roast at 400°F for 25-30 minutes. The chicken will be juicy, and the vegetables will be perfectly roasted for a balanced meal.
- **Salmon and Asparagus**: Place salmon fillets on one side of the sheet pan and asparagus spears on the other. Drizzle both with olive oil, lemon juice, and a sprinkle of garlic powder. Roast at 400°F for 15-20 minutes until the salmon is cooked through and the asparagus is tender. This simple meal is rich in omega-3 fatty acids and vitamins.
- **Sausage and Roasted Vegetables**: Slice chicken sausage (or your favorite sausage) and arrange it on a baking sheet with diced sweet potatoes, bell peppers, and Brussels sprouts. Drizzle with olive oil and season with paprika, salt, and pepper. Roast at 425°F for 20-25 minutes. The combination of savory sausage and caramelized vegetables makes this a hearty and flavorful dinner.
- **Pesto Chicken and Veggies**: Toss chicken breasts with pesto sauce and arrange them on a sheet pan with zucchini, cherry tomatoes, and red onion. Roast at 375°F for 25 minutes until the chicken is cooked through. This colorful, Mediterranean-inspired meal is packed with flavor and requires minimal effort.

Sheet pan dinners are great for meal prepping as well—simply double the recipe and store leftovers for lunch the next day.

One-Pot Pasta Recipes

One-pot pasta recipes are not only convenient but also incredibly flavorful, as the pasta absorbs the flavors of the ingredients while cooking. Here are some quick and delicious one-pot pasta ideas:

- **One-Pot Spinach and Tomato Pasta**: In a large pot, combine whole wheat pasta, cherry tomatoes, fresh spinach, garlic, and vegetable broth. Cook until the pasta is tender and the spinach is wilted. Stir in a splash of cream or sprinkle with Parmesan cheese for a rich and creamy finish.
- **Creamy Chicken Alfredo Pasta**: Cook pasta in a large pot with chicken broth and garlic. Once the pasta is almost done, add cooked chicken and a splash of cream or milk. Stir in Parmesan cheese and fresh parsley for a creamy, comforting dish that's ready in under 30 minutes.
- **Lemon Garlic Shrimp Pasta**: Cook pasta in a large pot with garlic and vegetable broth. Once the pasta is almost done, add shrimp, lemon zest, and a splash of lemon juice.

Cook until the shrimp are pink and the pasta is tender. Finish with fresh parsley and a drizzle of olive oil for a light and zesty meal.

- **One-Pot Pesto Pasta with Veggies**: Combine whole wheat pasta with zucchini, cherry tomatoes, garlic, and vegetable broth in a large pot. Cook until the pasta is tender, then stir in your favorite pesto sauce. Top with grated Parmesan cheese for a flavorful, veggie-packed dinner.

One-pot pasta meals save time on both cooking and clean-up, making them a perfect weeknight option.

Healthy Tacos and Wraps

Tacos and wraps are quick, customizable, and perfect for a busy evening. Here are some healthy taco and wrap ideas that come together in no time:

- **Fish Tacos with Cabbage Slaw**: Use grilled or baked white fish (such as cod or tilapia) as the base for these tacos. Top with a crunchy cabbage slaw made from shredded cabbage, lime juice, and cilantro. Serve in soft corn tortillas with a drizzle of yogurt-based sauce for a light yet flavorful dinner.
- **Chicken Fajita Wraps**: Sauté chicken breast strips with bell peppers, onions, and fajita seasoning. Serve the mixture in whole-wheat tortillas with a dollop of Greek yogurt and a sprinkle of cheese. These wraps are loaded with protein and veggies, making them a nutritious option for a quick dinner.
- **Black Bean and Sweet Potato Tacos**: Roast diced sweet potatoes with cumin and chili powder. Serve in soft tortillas with black beans, avocado, and a sprinkle of feta cheese. These vegetarian tacos are rich in fiber, protein, and healthy fats.
- **Turkey and Avocado Wraps**: Use sliced turkey breast, mashed avocado, lettuce, and tomato to create a simple, protein-packed wrap. Add a drizzle of mustard or a spread of hummus for extra flavor. Wrap it up in a whole-wheat tortilla for a satisfying and portable dinner.

Tacos and wraps can be made in advance or assembled quickly, making them a great option for busy evenings when you want something healthy yet delicious.

Chapter 7: Vegetarian Recipes in 30 Minutes or Less

Hearty Veggie Stir-Fries

Vegetarian stir-fries are a fantastic option for a quick, nutrient-packed meal. They are easily customizable and allow for the inclusion of various vegetables, plant-based proteins, and flavorful sauces. Here are some stir-fry ideas:

- **Tofu and Vegetable Stir-Fry**: Stir-fry firm tofu cubes with broccoli, bell peppers, and carrots in sesame oil. Add a sauce made from soy sauce, garlic, ginger, and a touch of maple syrup. Serve with brown rice or quinoa for a satisfying, protein-rich meal.
- **Mushroom and Bok Choy Stir-Fry**: Sauté sliced mushrooms with garlic, ginger, and bok choy. Add a splash of soy sauce and sesame oil for a quick and easy dish that's rich in vitamins and minerals. Serve with jasmine rice for a complete meal.
- **Peanut Sauce Veggie Stir-Fry**: Combine zucchini, bell peppers, carrots, and baby corn in a hot skillet. Toss the vegetables in a homemade peanut sauce made from peanut butter, soy sauce, lime juice, and a touch of Sriracha. This creamy, spicy stir-fry is perfect for a quick, plant-based dinner.
- **Chickpea and Spinach Stir-Fry**: Sauté chickpeas with spinach, garlic, and onion in olive oil. Add cumin and paprika for extra flavor, and serve over couscous or quinoa. This dish is packed with protein and fiber, making it a filling and nutritious meal.

Stir-fries are quick, healthy, and versatile, allowing you to use whatever vegetables you have on hand.

Vegetarian Pasta Dishes

Pasta dishes are another great option for quick vegetarian meals. By incorporating vegetables and plant-based proteins, you can create hearty, balanced meals in under 30 minutes. Here are a few ideas:

- **Zucchini and Tomato Pasta**: Sauté zucchini and cherry tomatoes with garlic in olive oil. Toss with whole wheat pasta and top with Parmesan cheese and fresh basil for a simple yet flavorful meal. This dish is light, healthy, and full of fresh flavors.
- **Creamy Spinach and Mushroom Pasta**: Sauté mushrooms and spinach in garlic and olive oil. Add a splash of cream or plant-based milk and stir in cooked whole wheat pasta. Top with a sprinkle of Parmesan or nutritional yeast for a creamy, comforting pasta dish that's rich in iron and fiber.
- **Lemon Garlic Broccoli Pasta**: Cook pasta in a large pot of salted water. In a separate pan, sauté broccoli with garlic, olive oil, and red pepper flakes. Toss the pasta with the broccoli and finish with a squeeze of lemon juice for a zesty, light meal.
- **Pesto and Veggie Pasta**: Toss cooked pasta with sautéed bell peppers, cherry tomatoes, and zucchini. Stir in your favorite pesto sauce and top with toasted pine nuts or sunflower seeds. This veggie-packed pasta dish is bursting with flavor and nutrients.

Pasta dishes are easy to adapt based on your preferences, and they can be prepared quickly with minimal ingredients.

Vegetarian One-Pot Meals

One-pot meals are convenient, requiring fewer dishes and making clean-up easier. Here are some vegetarian one-pot meal ideas that you can prepare in under 30 minutes:

- **One-Pot Lentil Curry**: In a large pot, sauté onions, garlic, and ginger with curry powder. Add lentils, diced tomatoes, and coconut milk. Simmer until the lentils are tender, and serve with brown rice or naan bread. This hearty, flavorful dish is rich in protein and perfect for meal prep.
- **Chickpea and Spinach Stew**: In a large pot, sauté onions and garlic in olive oil. Add canned chickpeas, diced tomatoes, and vegetable broth. Stir in fresh spinach and season with cumin, paprika, and chili flakes. Serve with crusty bread or over quinoa for a filling, nutrient-dense meal.
- **One-Pot Vegetable Soup**: Combine carrots, celery, zucchini, tomatoes, and spinach in a large pot with vegetable broth. Add garlic, thyme, and bay leaves for flavor. Simmer until the vegetables are tender, and serve with a side of whole-grain bread for a light yet hearty dinner.
- **One-Pot Pasta Primavera**: In a large pot, cook pasta with vegetable broth, garlic, and cherry tomatoes. Once the pasta is almost done, add asparagus, zucchini, and spinach. Stir in Parmesan cheese or nutritional yeast for a creamy, veggie-packed pasta dish that's perfect for a quick weeknight dinner.

One-pot meals are ideal for busy evenings and meal prepping, as they are easy to make and store well.

Vegetarian Tacos and Wraps

Tacos and wraps make for quick, customizable vegetarian dinners. Here are some ideas for tasty plant-based tacos and wraps:

- **Black Bean and Avocado Tacos**: Fill soft corn tortillas with black beans, sliced avocado, and a sprinkle of cotija cheese. Top with salsa and fresh cilantro for a simple, protein-packed taco that's ready in minutes.
- **Sweet Potato and Black Bean Wrap**: Roast diced sweet potatoes with cumin and chili powder, then combine them with black beans, shredded lettuce, and avocado in a whole-wheat wrap. This hearty, flavorful wrap is rich in fiber and healthy fats.
- **Chickpea Shawarma Wrap**: Toss roasted chickpeas with cumin, paprika, and garlic powder. Serve in a whole-wheat pita with lettuce, cucumber, tomato, and a drizzle of tahini sauce for a Middle Eastern-inspired wrap that's full of flavor.
- **Grilled Veggie Tacos**: Grill bell peppers, zucchini, and onions, and serve them in soft tortillas with a sprinkle of feta cheese and a drizzle of yogurt-based sauce. These tacos are light, healthy, and bursting with fresh flavors.

Vegetarian tacos and wraps are quick to prepare and offer endless possibilities for customization based on your preferences.

Chapter 8: Snacks and Sides in 30 Minutes or Less

Healthy Dips and Spreads

Wholesome dips and spreads are a great way to add flavor to snacks or serve as sides for meals. These options are nutrient-dense and can be prepared quickly.

- **Classic Hummus**: Blend canned chickpeas, tahini, olive oil, garlic, lemon juice, and a pinch of salt in a food processor until smooth. Serve with sliced veggies or whole-wheat pita bread for a high-protein, fiber-rich snack.
- **Guacamole**: Mash ripe avocados with lime juice, diced tomatoes, red onion, and cilantro. Add a pinch of salt and pepper for seasoning. Serve with baked tortilla chips or use as a spread for sandwiches and wraps.
- **Greek Yogurt Tzatziki**: Combine Greek yogurt with grated cucumber, garlic, lemon juice, and fresh dill. This light, tangy dip pairs perfectly with raw veggies, grilled meats, or as a side for wraps.
- **Spicy Black Bean Dip**: Blend canned black beans with garlic, lime juice, cumin, and a touch of chili powder. Serve with whole-grain crackers or veggie sticks for a protein-packed, spicy snack.

Dips and spreads are versatile and can be prepared in under 15 minutes, making them ideal for quick snacks or sides.

Quick Salad Sides

Salads are refreshing and light side dishes that can be prepared in minutes. These salad options are packed with nutrients and complement a variety of main meals:

- **Cucumber and Tomato Salad**: Toss sliced cucumbers, cherry tomatoes, and red onions with olive oil, lemon juice, and fresh herbs like parsley or mint. This simple, refreshing salad pairs well with grilled dishes or pasta.
- **Greek Salad**: Combine cucumbers, tomatoes, Kalamata olives, red onion, and feta cheese. Drizzle with olive oil and oregano for a flavorful Mediterranean side. This salad is rich in healthy fats and antioxidants.

- **Quinoa Tabbouleh**: Mix cooked quinoa with diced tomatoes, cucumbers, parsley, and mint. Add a lemon juice and olive oil dressing for a vibrant, nutrient-packed side. This salad can also be made in advance and stored for later meals.
- **Carrot and Raisin Salad**: Shred fresh carrots and mix with raisins, a splash of lemon juice, and a drizzle of honey. This lightly sweet, crunchy salad is a great side for sandwiches or wraps.

Salads are easy to customize based on your preferences and can be made quickly with minimal ingredients.

Simple Roasted Vegetables

Roasting vegetables is an easy way to enhance their natural sweetness and flavor. Here are a few quick and healthy roasted side dishes:

- **Roasted Sweet Potatoes**: Toss diced sweet potatoes with olive oil, cumin, and paprika. Roast at 400°F for 20-25 minutes until tender and caramelized. These make a delicious side for any main dish or can be added to salads and grain bowls.
- **Roasted Brussels Sprouts**: Slice Brussels sprouts in half and toss with olive oil, salt, and pepper. Roast at 425°F for 20 minutes until crispy. Add a drizzle of balsamic vinegar for extra flavor.
- **Roasted Carrots with Honey**: Toss baby carrots with olive oil and a drizzle of honey. Roast at 400°F for 20 minutes until tender and lightly caramelized. This sweet and savory side is a perfect accompaniment to grilled or baked proteins.
- **Garlic Roasted Cauliflower**: Toss cauliflower florets with olive oil, minced garlic, and a sprinkle of Parmesan cheese. Roast at 425°F for 20-25 minutes until golden brown. This crispy, flavorful side pairs well with pasta or grain dishes.

Roasted vegetables are simple to prepare and can be seasoned in various ways to suit your taste.

Easy-to-Make Snacks

Snacks that are both healthy and quick to prepare are great for busy days. Here are some snack ideas that you can make in under 30 minutes:

- **Energy Bites**: Combine rolled oats, peanut butter, honey, and chia seeds in a bowl. Roll into small balls and refrigerate for 15 minutes. These energy bites are rich in protein and make a great snack to grab on the go.
- **Apple and Nut Butter Slices**: Slice an apple and spread almond butter or peanut butter on top. Sprinkle with chia seeds or cinnamon for added flavor and nutrition. This snack is quick, simple, and full of healthy fats.
- **Veggie Sticks with Hummus**: Slice carrots, cucumbers, and bell peppers and serve with homemade or store-bought hummus. This crunchy snack is full of fiber and makes for a light yet satisfying snack.
- **Avocado Toast**: Mash half an avocado and spread it on whole-grain toast. Add a sprinkle of salt, pepper, and red pepper flakes for a delicious, nutrient-packed snack. Top with a poached egg for an extra boost of protein.

Snacks like these can be made quickly and are great for keeping your energy levels up throughout the day.

Chapter 9: Smoothies and Drinks in 30 Minutes or Less

Refreshing Fruit Smoothies

Smoothies are a quick and easy way to pack a lot of nutrition into one glass. Here are some refreshing fruit smoothie ideas that can be whipped up in minutes:

- **Berry Banana Smoothie**: Blend a banana with frozen mixed berries, a cup of Greek yogurt, and a splash of almond milk. This smoothie is rich in antioxidants, fiber, and protein, making it a great way to start the day or enjoy as a snack.
- **Mango Pineapple Smoothie**: Combine frozen mango chunks, pineapple, and coconut water in a blender. Add a handful of spinach for an extra boost of nutrients. This tropical smoothie is hydrating and full of vitamins A and C.
- **Peach and Oat Smoothie**: Blend a frozen peach with a handful of oats, almond milk, and a drizzle of honey. The oats add fiber and texture, making this smoothie both filling and delicious.
- **Watermelon Mint Smoothie**: Blend cubed watermelon with a handful of fresh mint leaves, lime juice, and ice. This hydrating, refreshing smoothie is perfect for hot days and is packed with vitamins and antioxidants.

Smoothies are endlessly customizable, allowing you to mix and match fruits, vegetables, and proteins based on your preferences.

Green Smoothies for an Energy Boost

Green smoothies are a great way to incorporate leafy greens like spinach or kale into your diet. These smoothies are packed with vitamins, minerals, and antioxidants:

- **Spinach and Apple Smoothie**: Blend fresh spinach with a green apple, banana, and a cup of almond milk. Add a teaspoon of chia seeds for extra fiber. This vibrant smoothie is refreshing and nutrient-dense, perfect for boosting energy.
- **Kale and Pineapple Smoothie**: Blend kale with frozen pineapple, coconut milk, and a small piece of ginger. This tropical smoothie is full of vitamins and has a refreshing, slightly spicy kick from the ginger.
- **Avocado Green Smoothie**: Blend half an avocado with spinach, banana, almond milk, and a tablespoon of flaxseeds. This creamy smoothie is rich in healthy fats and perfect for keeping you full throughout the day.
- **Cucumber and Mint Smoothie**: Blend cucumber, spinach, a handful of fresh mint, and a splash of lemon juice. This smoothie is hydrating, refreshing, and packed with vitamins. It's perfect for a light snack or to rehydrate after a workout.

Green smoothies are a simple way to boost your vegetable intake while enjoying a delicious and easy-to-make drink.

Protein-Packed Smoothies

Protein smoothies are perfect for refueling after a workout or keeping you satisfied between meals. Here are a few protein-rich smoothie options:

- **Peanut Butter Banana Protein Smoothie**: Blend a banana with a tablespoon of peanut butter, a scoop of vanilla protein powder, and a cup of almond milk. This smoothie is rich in protein and healthy fats, making it perfect for a post-workout snack.
- **Chocolate Protein Smoothie**: Blend a scoop of chocolate protein powder with frozen banana, almond milk, and a tablespoon of cocoa powder. Add a handful of spinach for extra nutrients. This smoothie tastes indulgent while still being packed with nutrition.
- **Almond Butter and Blueberry Smoothie**: Blend a handful of frozen blueberries with almond butter, a scoop of protein powder, and oat milk. This smoothie is rich in antioxidants and protein, making it perfect for breakfast or a snack.
- **Greek Yogurt Smoothie**: Blend Greek yogurt with frozen mixed berries, spinach, and a drizzle of honey. This smoothie is packed with protein and probiotics, making it a great option for gut health and keeping you full.

These protein-packed smoothies are ideal for busy days when you need a quick and nutritious meal or snack.

Healthy Homemade Drinks

Aside from smoothies, there are several easy-to-make drinks that are both refreshing and packed with health benefits. Here are a few ideas for homemade drinks that you can prepare quickly:

- **Lemon Ginger Detox Water**: Slice fresh lemons and ginger, then add them to a pitcher of water. Let it sit for 10-15 minutes for the flavors to infuse. This refreshing drink is great for hydration and digestion.
- **Iced Green Tea with Honey**: Brew green tea and let it cool. Add a teaspoon of honey and pour over ice. Green tea is full of antioxidants and makes a great afternoon pick-me-up.
- **Cucumber Mint Infused Water**: Add sliced cucumbers and fresh mint leaves to a pitcher of water. Let it sit for 10 minutes to infuse the flavors. This hydrating drink is refreshing and perfect for a hot day.
- **Chia Seed Lemonade**: Mix fresh lemon juice, water, and a tablespoon of chia seeds. Let the chia seeds sit for a few minutes until they absorb the water and form a gel-like consistency. This drink is full of fiber and a refreshing alternative to sugary beverages.

These homemade drinks are easy to prepare and can be enjoyed throughout the day for hydration and health benefits.

Chapter 10: Breakfast Recipes in 30 Minutes or Less

Quick and Nutritious Smoothie Bowls
Smoothie bowls are a fun twist on smoothies, offering a thicker consistency that you can enjoy with a spoon and topped with various toppings. They are colorful, nutritious, and perfect for breakfast:

- **Berry Smoothie Bowl**: Blend frozen mixed berries, banana, and Greek yogurt for a thick, creamy base. Top with granola, chia seeds, and fresh berries. This breakfast is packed with antioxidants, protein, and fiber.
- **Tropical Smoothie Bowl**: Blend frozen mango, pineapple, and coconut milk. Top with shredded coconut, sliced kiwi, and almonds. This tropical bowl is rich in vitamin C and healthy fats, making it a refreshing start to your day.
- **Green Smoothie Bowl**: Blend spinach, banana, and almond milk for a nutrient-packed green smoothie. Top with sliced strawberries, chia seeds, and a sprinkle of granola. This bowl is packed with vitamins, fiber, and healthy fats.
- **Chocolate Peanut Butter Smoothie Bowl**: Blend frozen banana, a tablespoon of peanut butter, cocoa powder, and almond milk for a rich and indulgent smoothie bowl. Top with crushed peanuts, sliced banana, and cacao nibs. This is a protein-packed, filling breakfast option.

Smoothie bowls are versatile, easy to make, and can be customized with your favorite toppings.

Healthy Breakfast Wraps
Breakfast wraps are a great way to combine protein, veggies, and healthy fats into a portable meal. Here are some quick and easy breakfast wrap ideas:

- **Scrambled Egg and Veggie Wrap**: Scramble eggs with spinach, tomatoes, and onions. Place in a whole wheat tortilla and sprinkle with shredded cheese. Roll it up for a quick, high-protein breakfast wrap.
- **Avocado and Black Bean Wrap**: Mash avocado and spread it on a whole wheat tortilla. Add black beans, scrambled eggs, and salsa. This wrap is full of fiber and healthy fats, making it a filling and nutritious breakfast.
- **Smoked Salmon Breakfast Wrap**: Spread cream cheese on a whole wheat tortilla and add smoked salmon, scrambled eggs, and fresh spinach. This wrap is rich in omega-3s, protein, and vitamins, making it a healthy breakfast option.
- **Peanut Butter and Banana Wrap**: Spread peanut butter on a whole wheat tortilla, add banana slices, and drizzle with honey. Roll it up for a quick, energy-boosting breakfast that's perfect for busy mornings.

These breakfast wraps are easy to make and can be enjoyed on the go, making them ideal for busy mornings.

Overnight Oats

Overnight oats are a no-cook breakfast option that you can prepare the night before and enjoy in the morning. They are nutritious, customizable, and take less than 5 minutes to prepare:

- **Classic Overnight Oats**: Combine rolled oats, almond milk, and a tablespoon of chia seeds in a jar. Let it sit in the fridge overnight, and in the morning, top with fresh berries, nuts, and a drizzle of honey. This fiber-rich breakfast is filling and easy to make.
- **Chocolate Peanut Butter Overnight Oats**: Mix rolled oats, almond milk, cocoa powder, and a tablespoon of peanut butter. Let it sit overnight and top with sliced bananas in the morning. This protein-packed breakfast is indulgent yet healthy.
- **Apple Cinnamon Overnight Oats**: Combine rolled oats, almond milk, cinnamon, and diced apples in a jar. Let it sit overnight, and top with a sprinkle of walnuts or almonds for extra crunch. This is a comforting, nutritious breakfast that's perfect for fall mornings.
- **Pumpkin Spice Overnight Oats**: Mix rolled oats, almond milk, canned pumpkin, and a dash of pumpkin pie spice. Let it sit overnight and top with pecans and a drizzle of maple syrup. This seasonal breakfast is rich in fiber and flavor.

Overnight oats are perfect for meal prep, as they can be made ahead of time and enjoyed throughout the week.

Quick and Healthy Pancakes

Pancakes can be made healthier with the right ingredients, and they don't have to take a long time to prepare. Here are some quick and healthy pancake options:

- **Banana Oat Pancakes**: Blend a banana, oats, eggs, and a dash of cinnamon in a blender. Cook in a skillet until golden brown. These pancakes are gluten-free and packed with fiber and protein.
- **Blueberry Whole Wheat Pancakes**: Mix whole wheat flour, baking powder, almond milk, and fresh blueberries. Cook in a non-stick skillet for a healthy twist on classic pancakes that are rich in antioxidants and fiber.
- **Almond Flour Pancakes**: Combine almond flour, eggs, baking powder, and a splash of vanilla extract. These low-carb, high-protein pancakes are perfect for a quick and healthy breakfast.
- **Pumpkin Pancakes**: Mix canned pumpkin, eggs, whole wheat flour, and a dash of cinnamon. These pancakes are rich in fiber and vitamins, making them a nutritious and filling breakfast option.

These pancake recipes are easy to prepare, nutritious, and can be made in under 30 minutes for a wholesome breakfast.

Chapter 11: Meal Prep Tips for Quick Cooking

1. Plan Your Meals Ahead

Planning is key to effective meal prep. Set aside some time each week to decide what meals you want to prepare. Here are some tips to help you get started:

- **Create a Weekly Menu**: Write down a simple menu for the week, including breakfast, lunch, dinner, and snacks. This will help you stay organized and ensure you have all the ingredients on hand.
- **Choose Recipes Wisely**: Select recipes that use similar ingredients. This will help reduce waste and save you time shopping and prepping.
- **Keep It Simple**: Choose quick and easy recipes that you can prepare in 30 minutes or less. Focus on meals that require minimal cooking and use simple cooking techniques.
- **Consider Leftovers**: Plan for meals that will leave you with leftovers. This can save time on days when you're too busy to cook.

2. Make a Grocery List

Once you've planned your meals, create a detailed grocery list based on the ingredients you'll need. Here are some tips for effective shopping:

- **Organize by Category**: Sort your grocery list by category (produce, dairy, grains, etc.) to make shopping more efficient.
- **Check Your Pantry**: Before heading to the store, check what you already have in your pantry and refrigerator. This will help prevent unnecessary purchases.
- **Stick to the List**: Try to stick to your grocery list to avoid impulse buys. This will save you time and money.

3. Pre-Chop and Prep Ingredients

Prepping ingredients ahead of time can significantly cut down on cooking time during the week. Here's how to streamline your prep:

- **Wash and Chop Vegetables**: Wash and chop vegetables like bell peppers, carrots, and cucumbers. Store them in airtight containers in the fridge for easy access.
- **Cook Grains in Batches**: Cook large batches of grains like rice, quinoa, or farro. Store them in the fridge to use throughout the week in various meals.
- **Pre-portion Snacks**: Portion out snacks like nuts, fruits, or veggie sticks into grab-and-go containers. This will help you stay on track with healthy eating.
- **Prepare Sauces and Dressings**: Make sauces and dressings in advance and store them in jars. Having these on hand can add flavor to meals quickly.

4. Invest in Quality Storage Containers

Having the right storage containers can make a big difference in your meal prep experience. Here are some tips for choosing the right containers:

- **Opt for Glass Containers**: Glass containers are durable, microwave-safe, and great for reheating leftovers. They are also less likely to retain odors compared to plastic containers.
- **Use BPA-free Plastic Containers**: If you prefer plastic, make sure to choose BPA-free options that are microwave and dishwasher safe.
- **Consider Portion Control**: Use containers that are portioned for specific meals or snacks. This can help with portion control and prevent overeating.
- **Label and Date Your Containers**: Use labels to mark what's inside each container and the date it was prepared. This helps keep your meals organized and ensures you eat them while they're fresh.

5. Cook in Batches

Batch cooking is an effective strategy for saving time in the kitchen. Here's how to incorporate batch cooking into your routine:

- **Cook Large Portions**: Prepare large portions of meals that freeze well, such as soups, stews, and casseroles. Portion them out and freeze for easy meals later.
- **Utilize One-Pot Meals**: One-pot meals are perfect for batch cooking, as they often yield multiple servings and require minimal clean-up.
- **Double Your Recipes**: When cooking a dish, consider doubling the recipe. You can enjoy the leftovers for lunch or dinner the next day, or freeze them for later.
- **Use Slow Cookers or Instant Pots**: These appliances are great for batch cooking, as they allow you to set it and forget it. Prepare ingredients in the morning, and come home to a hot, ready meal.

6. Embrace Freezer-Friendly Meals

Freezing meals can be a lifesaver for busy weeks. Here are some freezer-friendly options to consider:

- **Soups and Stews**: Most soups and stews freeze well. Make a big batch and freeze individual portions for quick reheating.
- **Cooked Grains**: Cooked rice, quinoa, and pasta can be frozen in portions and easily reheated.
- **Marinated Proteins**: Marinate chicken, fish, or tofu and freeze them in individual portions. Thaw and cook as needed for quick meals.
- **Smoothie Packs**: Prepare smoothie bags by portioning out fruits and greens in freezer bags. Just blend with your choice of liquid in the morning for a quick breakfast.

7. Organize Your Kitchen

An organized kitchen can streamline your cooking process. Here's how to keep your space tidy:

- **Keep Essentials Within Reach**: Store frequently used items, like spices and cooking oils, within easy reach. This can save time when you're in the middle of cooking.
- **Use Clear Storage Bins**: Use clear bins to organize snacks, pantry staples, and meal prep items. This makes it easy to find what you need quickly.

- **Label Shelves and Containers**: Labeling can help you quickly identify where everything is and keep your kitchen tidy.
- **Maintain a Clean Workspace**: Regularly clean and declutter your kitchen to make cooking more enjoyable and efficient.

8. Set a Cooking Schedule

Designate specific days and times for meal prep to make it a regular part of your routine. Here's how to establish a cooking schedule:

- **Choose a Prep Day**: Pick one day a week, such as Sunday, for your meal prep. Dedicate a couple of hours to prepare meals and snacks for the week ahead.
- **Incorporate Quick Cooking Days**: On days when you have more time, try to prepare larger batches or more elaborate meals.
- **Involve Family Members**: Get family members involved in the meal prep process. Cooking together can make it more enjoyable and efficient.

By incorporating these meal prep tips into your routine, you can save time, reduce stress, and ensure that you always have healthy meals on hand.

Chapter 12: Quick Cooking Techniques for Busy People

1. One-Pan and One-Pot Meals

One-pan and one-pot meals are a lifesaver for busy individuals. These cooking methods minimize clean-up while allowing you to prepare delicious and nutritious meals quickly. Here's how to make the most of these techniques:

- **Sheet Pan Dinners**: Toss protein (such as chicken, fish, or tofu) and an assortment of vegetables with olive oil and your favorite seasonings. Spread everything on a sheet pan and roast in the oven until cooked through, usually about 20-30 minutes. This method allows for easy cleanup and minimizes the number of dishes used.
- **One-Pot Pasta**: Combine pasta, vegetables, broth, and seasonings in a single pot. Cook according to package instructions, allowing the pasta to absorb the flavors as it cooks. This technique yields a flavorful dish with minimal cleanup.
- **Skillet Meals**: Sauté your protein and vegetables in a large skillet with a bit of oil. Add cooked grains or pasta to the skillet and toss everything together with your choice of sauce or seasoning. This method allows for quick cooking and easy flavor customization.
- **Slow Cooker and Instant Pot Meals**: These appliances are excellent for busy days. You can prep your ingredients in the morning, set the timer, and come home to a ready meal. Slow cookers work well for soups, stews, and casseroles, while Instant Pots can prepare grains and proteins in a fraction of the time.

2. Blanching and Freezing Vegetables

Blanching is a quick cooking technique that preserves the color, flavor, and nutrients of vegetables. This method involves briefly boiling vegetables and then immediately placing them in ice water. Here's how to do it:

- **Choose Your Vegetables**: Select fresh vegetables like broccoli, green beans, or carrots for blanching.
- **Prepare Ice Bath**: Fill a bowl with ice and cold water. This will stop the cooking process after blanching.
- **Blanch the Vegetables**: Boil water in a large pot and add the vegetables for 1-3 minutes, depending on the vegetable. After blanching, quickly transfer the vegetables to the ice bath to cool them down.
- **Store for Later Use**: Drain the vegetables and pat them dry. Store in airtight containers or freezer bags to keep them fresh for future meals. Blanched vegetables can be added to stir-fries, salads, or served as sides with minimal cooking required.

3. Use Pre-Cooked Ingredients

Utilizing pre-cooked or pre-prepared ingredients can significantly speed up your cooking process. Here are some tips:

- **Rotisserie Chicken**: Purchase a rotisserie chicken from the store for quick meals. Use it in salads, sandwiches, wraps, or as a main dish paired with your favorite sides.
- **Pre-Cooked Grains**: Look for pre-cooked rice, quinoa, or other grains available at the grocery store. These can be heated quickly and used as a base for various meals.
- **Frozen Vegetables**: Frozen vegetables are a convenient option that can be quickly added to stir-fries, soups, or casseroles without the need for washing and chopping.
- **Canned Legumes**: Canned beans and lentils are ready to use and can be added to salads, soups, or grain bowls for a protein boost. Rinse them under cold water to reduce sodium content before using.

4. Quick Cooking Methods

Familiarizing yourself with quick cooking methods can help you prepare meals faster. Here are some techniques to incorporate into your cooking:

- **Sautéing**: This method involves cooking food quickly over high heat with a small amount of oil. It's perfect for vegetables and proteins, as it retains flavor and texture.
- **Stir-Frying**: Similar to sautéing, stir-frying involves cooking small pieces of food quickly in a hot wok or skillet. The high heat helps seal in flavors and nutrients, making it an excellent technique for quick meals.

- **Grilling**: Grilling can be done indoors or outdoors and is a quick way to cook proteins and vegetables. Use a grill pan or an outdoor grill for quick cooking that adds great flavor.
- **Microwaving**: Don't underestimate the power of your microwave! Use it to quickly steam vegetables, heat grains, or even cook certain proteins. It's an excellent option for busy mornings when time is of the essence.

5. Mastering the Art of Meal Assembly

Sometimes, the fastest meals come from assembling rather than cooking. Here are some ideas for quick meal assembly:

- **Grain Bowls**: Start with a base of cooked grains (like rice or quinoa) and top with your choice of protein, vegetables, and sauces. This versatile meal is easy to customize and can be made quickly.
- **Wraps and Sandwiches**: Use whole grain wraps or bread and fill them with deli meats, cheese, veggies, and spreads. These can be put together in minutes and are perfect for lunch or a light dinner.
- **Salad Kits**: Keep pre-washed salad greens and a variety of toppings on hand for quick salads. Combine greens with proteins, nuts, seeds, and dressings for a nutritious meal.
- **Snack Plates**: Assemble snack plates with a variety of items like hummus, cheese, nuts, fruits, and whole grain crackers. These can serve as quick meals or satisfying snacks.

6. Optimize Your Time in the Kitchen

Efficiently using your time in the kitchen can make meal preparation quicker and more enjoyable. Here are some tips for optimizing your cooking time:

- **Prep Ingredients First**: Before cooking, gather and prep all your ingredients. This makes the cooking process smoother and faster.
- **Clean as You Go**: Keep your workspace tidy by cleaning up as you cook. This will save you time on cleanup at the end.
- **Use a Timer**: Set a timer for each cooking step to keep yourself on track. This helps you stay focused and can speed up your cooking process.
- **Involve Others**: If possible, involve family members or friends in meal prep. Assign tasks to make the process faster and more enjoyable.

By incorporating these quick cooking techniques into your routine, you can save time and make healthy cooking more accessible, even on your busiest days.

Conclusion

In today's fast-paced world, finding time to prepare healthy meals can often feel like a daunting task. However, with the right strategies and techniques, you can create nutritious and delicious meals in just 30 minutes or less. Throughout this book, we have explored a variety of quick recipes, meal prep tips, and cooking techniques designed to help you make the most of your time in the kitchen.

By planning your meals, utilizing pre-cooked ingredients, and mastering quick cooking methods, you can streamline your cooking process and maintain a healthy lifestyle. Remember, the key to successful meal prep is consistency and creativity. Don't be afraid to experiment with new flavors and ingredients to keep your meals exciting.

As you embark on your journey to quick and healthy cooking, remember that every small change you make can lead to a healthier, more balanced life. Enjoy the process, share your meals with loved ones, and embrace the joy of cooking.

Thank you for choosing **"30-Minute Meal Prep: Quick and Healthy Recipes for Busy People."** May your kitchen be filled with flavor, and your table surrounded by those you love.

Acknowledgments

I would like to express my heartfelt gratitude to everyone who has supported me throughout this journey of creating **"30-Minute Meal Prep: Quick and Healthy Recipes for Busy People."**

First and foremost, thank you to my family and friends for your unwavering encouragement and belief in my vision. Your enthusiasm for my recipes and your willingness to taste-test my creations inspired me to bring this book to life.

A special thanks to my mentor and culinary guide, whose invaluable advice and expertise helped shape my cooking skills and approach to meal prep. Your insights have been instrumental in my development as a cook and writer.

To all the chefs, food bloggers, and nutritionists whose work has inspired me, thank you for sharing your knowledge and passion for healthy cooking. Your creativity and dedication have influenced my recipes and cooking philosophy.

Finally, I extend my appreciation to you, the reader. Your interest in quick and healthy cooking drives my desire to create, and I hope this book serves you well on your culinary journey.

Resources Section

Here are some additional resources to help you on your meal prep journey:

1. Meal Prep Websites and Blogs

- **Minimalist Baker**: A fantastic resource for simple, healthy recipes with a focus on whole foods.
- **EatingWell**: Offers a wide variety of meal prep ideas and recipes that emphasize nutrition and flavor.
- **Fit Foodie Finds**: Features healthy meal prep recipes, tips, and ideas for busy lifestyles.

2. Meal Prep Cookbooks

- **"Meal Prep for Beginners" by Michelle D. McGann**: A great starting point for those new to meal prepping.
- **"The Meal Prep King Plan" by Meal Prep King**: This book offers a comprehensive approach to meal prep with a variety of recipes.
- **"Preppy Kitchen" by John Kanell**: Focuses on meal prep with delicious recipes and practical tips.

3. Kitchen Tools and Gadgets

- **Food Processor**: Ideal for chopping vegetables and making sauces quickly.
- **Instant Pot**: A versatile tool for pressure cooking, slow cooking, and meal prep.
- **Glass Meal Prep Containers**: Durable and microwave-safe, perfect for storing prepped meals.

4. Online Cooking Classes

- **MasterClass**: Offers cooking classes from renowned chefs, providing valuable insights and techniques.
- **Udemy**: Features various online courses on meal prep and cooking for different skill levels.

5. Nutrition Resources

- **ChooseMyPlate.gov**: Provides guidelines on balanced meals and portion control.
- **Nutrition.gov**: Offers reliable information on nutrition and healthy eating practices.

www.ingramcontent.com/pod-product-compliance
Lightning Source LLC
Chambersburg PA
CBHW081637250726
48657CB00009B/2931